# HOMEOPATHY

by
Christopher Day
MA, VetMB, MRCVS, VetFFHom, CertIAVH

Illustrations by
Carole Vincer

KENILWORTH PRESS

First published in Great Britain by
The Kenilworth Press Limited,
Addington, Buckingham, MK18 2JR

© The Kenilworth Press Limited, 2000

**British Library Cataloguing in Publication Data**
A catalogue record for this book is available from the British Library.

ISBN 1-872119-24-7

Printed in Great Britain by Westway Offset, Wembley

**The Law: UK Legislation Relevant to This Booklet**
Veterinary Surgeons Act, 1966; Medicines Act, 1968; Cruelty to Animals Act, 1911

The implication of this legislation is that only a qualified veterinary
surgeon may legally treat or prescribe for your horse. There are many
non-veterinarians who set out to treat horses and it is an unfortunate
sequel to the Veterinary Surgeons Act that, if an owner consults a non-
vet and thereby fails to alleviate suffering for his or her animal,
prosecution under the 1911 Act is a possibility.

Also, it is worth studying Food Labelling legislation, which will aid
in understanding the declared ingredients on horse feeds and
supplement labels.

# Contents

# Introduction

In these days of burgeoning interest in all things natural and holistic, the demand for homeopathic care for horses is understandably and rightly on the increase. Along with this increase, goes a thirst for greater knowledge and understanding of homeopathic theory, philosophy and methods, on the part of intelligent horse people.

An integral part of the modern move into natural medicine is a growing concern that modern drug medicine is not always safe and an understanding that the body has immense healing powers to correct its own health problems, given the right stimulus. The proper use of homeopathic medicines provides just the safe, gentle and effective stimulus required to bring about healing, in most cases of horse illness.

The purpose of this book is to equip the reader to treat many minor ailments in the stable, cheaply and effectively. It is also structured to show the scope of homeopathic treatment in the wider field of more serious disease, and how to obtain professional help in such situations.

The author is a practising veterinarian, who runs a referral practice for all forms of 'alternative', natural, holistic medicine. He travels widely in the UK, treating horses with all manner of health and locomotor problems. He is also a teacher of homeopathic veterinary medicine in the UK and worldwide.

# The Law

Certain restrictions can apply to home treatment and it is up to you to ensure that what you do is permitted in your state or country. In the UK, for example, it is illegal for a non-vet to provide treatment or diagnosis. This applies to herbs, acupuncture, Bach flowers, tissue salts, aromatherapy, anthroposophy or homeopathy and the law is quite clear on this (Veterinary Surgeons Act 1966). Exceptions are made for chiropractors, osteopaths and physiotherapists, who may all practise their specialities under veterinary supervision.

This means that in the UK you can give homeopathic treatment to horses under your care. Only veterinarians may do so for another person's horse, whether or not fees are requested. If a non-vet is consulted, no indemnity insurance is available.

Furthermore, if something were to go wrong, both the owner and the prescriber may be liable to prosecution under animal welfare legislation.

Readers are advised to be very wary of accepting the advice and products of those individuals or manufacturers who bend these rules for gain. It is dangerous to use non-professional advice, or to use herbs, homeopathy or other medicines offered by anyone who has not properly examined the patient. In Britain members of the BAHVS (British Association of Homeopathic Veterinary Surgeons) have signed up to a 'code of conduct' on this point.

# History

Homeopathy emerged as an effective healing force in the latter part of the eighteenth century. A German physician, Samuel Hahnemann (1755-1843), discovered that Cinchona Bark (which gives us Quinine) was a very effective medicine to treat malaria, simply because it was able to produce symptoms very similar to malaria when given to a healthy body.

Hahnemann was without the benefit of laboratories, in those days, for conducting experiments, so he used himself, family, friends and volunteers to test his theories. What emerged from his painstaking and very scientific work was the theory that 'like can cure like'. In other words, a substance that causes symptoms in a healthy body cures similar symptoms in a diseased patient.

After making this ground-breaking discovery, Hahnemann went on to experiment with extreme dilutions, in order to render his medicines totally safe. This work gave him his second surprise, revealing that, as he methodically diluted and violently agitated his medicines, he produced both increasing safety and increasing curative power. He called the latter 'potency'.

A great many medicines were 'proven' in this way by Hahnemann and his successors, and they were applied to animals, notably by Boenninghausen, in the early nineteenth century. To illustrate the power of homeopathy to cure even serious disease, it is worth noting that homoeopaths were able to cure those eighteenth-century scourges of typhus and cholera, well before science discovered bacteria or formulated germ theory!

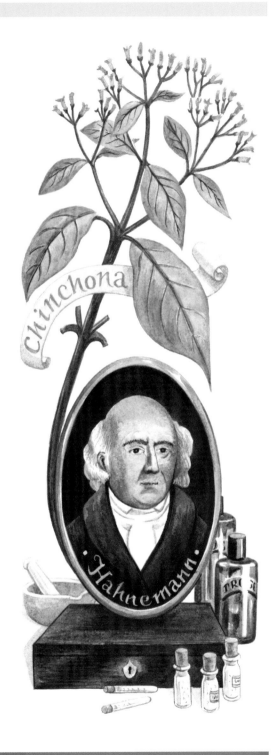

# Advantages of using homeopathy

Since properly applied homeopathy, supported by holistic diet, saddling, shoeing and management support, is able to tackle so many serious and worrying diseases with a good hope of success in most cases, it stands to reason that there are many advantages attached to its use. A few are mentioned here.

Homeopathic medicine is totally safe for any animal, but this is particularly important in the case of pregnant or lactating mares. No harm will come to foetus or foal at foot, as a result of judiciously prescribed homeopathic medicine.

Homeopathic medicines will never interfere with subsequent or intercurrent conventional drugs, given by your veterinary surgeon. This means that home medication is a serious possibility in many cases of illness, when the carer has the skill and knowledge to prescribe.

In competition horses, there is no fear of falling foul of any 'doping' rules. The extreme dilutions of homeopathic medicines mean that there can be no tissue or blood residues and, since we are only stimulating the healthy norm, or optimum, there can be no moral objection to its use either. Supernormal performance is not achievable with homeopathic medicines. The result of this is that, in a ringworm outbreak for instance, in an active racing or competition yard, the affected horses can be treated for the problem, cheaply and effectively, while 'in-contacts' are given preventive doses, all without anxieties about competition rules. Welfare objectives can be achieved in short time spans, while active participation by non-contagious horses can continue uninterrupted.

Under EU legislation, horses are classed as food animals. This means that there can be restrictions imposed on the use of conventional drugs under certain circumstances. Homeopathy is free from such constraints.

In most cases of disease, homeopathic medicines prove much cheaper than manufactured drug treatments. This is not the noblest reason for the use of homeopathy but it can be a powerful consideration in serious illness, when bills can mount up.

There are some diseases (mostly outside the scope of this book) for which there is no suitable conventional treatment. In these cases, homeopathy can often offer a realistic prospect. Cushing's disease, equine influenza and viral diseases in general present some examples of this; navicular disease, sinusitis, strangles, colic and many other troublesome diseases can also respond well. In addition, the resolution of more 'basic' disease, such as septic wounds, tendon injuries, sprains and arthritis can all be accelerated and improved by correct homeopathic prescribing.

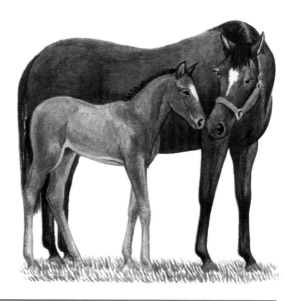

# Use and care of the remedies

Homeopathic medicines are very delicate, so it is essential to observe certain precautions in their use.

- **Do not handle them**, but give directly into the mouth or in a small portion of organic carrot or apple.

- **Do not give with hard feed,** preferably not feeding within half an hour.

- **Do not expose them to sunlight, extreme heat or frost.** Store remedies in an airtight brown glass container, in a cool, dark, cupboard. Do not refrigerate them.

- **Strong aromas can destroy them.** Do not give concurrent aromatherapy, unless under the supervision of a vet experienced in both therapies.

Homeopathic medicines are available in many different forms, to suit each situation.

As a general rule, a **dose** of a homeopathic medicine can be considered as:

- **four tablets**
- **six pillules**
- **one portion of powders or crystals** or
- **three or four drops of tincture**

The optimum frequency of dosing depends upon the severity and rapidity of the disease or condition. In **acute,** severe disease like colic, doses can be given every few minutes until relief is obtained. In the case of slow, **chronic** disease, intervals can be much greater, or even a single dose may suffice, awaiting responses over the coming weeks.

Creams, ointments or lotions are also available for topical use. These should be applied twice daily, unless directed otherwise by a veterinary surgeon.

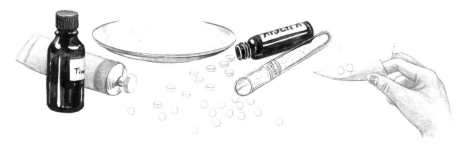

# Calling the vet

Knowing when to call for veterinary advice is always difficult. As a general rule: **when in doubt, call the vet.** It is usually safe to wait and see in non-dangerous, slow-onset conditions but not in the case of acute, severe illness. Colic is one such example. It is usually safer to call the vet in all such cases. It is quite reasonable, however, while awaiting the vet's arrival, to give doses of a well-chosen homeopathic medicine. If the

vet is delayed, your medicine could prove invaluable. In some cases, a cure may even be achieved before the vet arrives. At no time will the remedy ever interfere with a vet's treatment.

If ever you do treat your own horse and subsequently call in a vet, be sure to tell the vet what you have done. This is always constructive.

# Treatment guide for common ailments

Only the simplest conditions are listed here, since this is a guide for beginners. In all circumstances of doubt or of failed therapy, call a veterinary surgeon.

*Unless otherwise specified, it is intended that these medicines should be given by mouth, either as pills or tablets, or as liquids.*

## Abuse

*This is, sadly, a common enough problem to warrant inclusion. Homeopathy has much to offer in such cases.*

 *Staphisagria* – this medicine can help enormously both in mental and physical recovery.

## Abrasions/grazes

 *Calendula lotion* – use on the affected area. It speeds healing and helps prevent infection.

 *Hypericum and Calendula lotion* – this is invaluable in painful cases.

*Hepar sulph.* – by mouth, in addition, if there is already infection.

## Aggression

*Arsen. alb.* – if this fails, a homeopathic vet may be able to help.

## Anxiety – see Nervousness

## Abscess

 *Belladonna* – if very painful, red and hot.

*Calc. sulph.* – if discharging but not healing.

 *Hepar sulph.* – if painful, yet not ready to burst.

*Silica* – if result of penetrating foreign body or if chronic.

 *Ledum* – in early stages, after a puncture wound, in an attempt to prevent infection.

## Arthritis

 *Rhus tox.* – if stiff on starting to move, then loosens up.

*Bryonia* – if worse for any movement, or for continued movement.

 *Calc. fluor.* – if bony distortion of joints.

*Causticum* – if worse in bright frosty weather.

 *Ruta grav.* – if joint capsules or cartilage are affected.

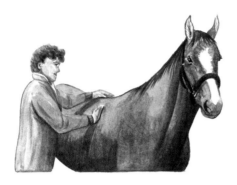

## Back problems

*Rhus tox., Ruta grav. and Arnica –* use these in combination for first aid. Seek veterinary help if complicated.

*The author uses chiropractic techniques to correct misalignment. Massage can also be very useful. The saddle and shoeing should also be checked very carefully. These measures are important, if recovery is to be optimised. The horse should not be ridden until comfortable.*

## Bereavement – see Pining

## Bites

*Hypericum and Calendula lotion –* use topically, to aid healing.

### • from other horses

*Arnica –* to help with the bruising.

*Hepar sulph. –* if infected.

### • bites and stings by insects

*Apis mel. –* if swollen.

*Cantharis –* if blistered.

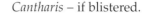
*Urtica –* if urticarial (nettle-rash type) reaction.

### • by snake – *call for veterinary help promptly but give:*

*Lachesis –* to try to reduce both the local tissue damage and the systemic effects of the poison. It is most suitable if the lesion tends to purple.

## Bone injury

*Arnica –* always helps to heal the bruising damage.

*Symphytum –* speeds and strengthens bone healing.

*Ruta grav. –* helps injured periosteum (membrane surrounding bone) to heal.

## Bruising

*Arnica –* this medicine is one of homeopathy's seeming miracles. It will always help in **any** case of injury, whether to horse or to rider, and its ability to reduce bruising, especially if given immediately after the injury, is legendary.

# Treatment guide cont.

## Burns and scalds

*Arnica* – to reduce swelling and pain.

*Cantharis* – to reduce or resolve blistering.

*Cantharis lotion* – this will be very healing and restorative, if applied to the area.

## Chilling

*Aconite* – this remedy is always indicated where there is sudden disruption of mental or physical equilibrium. It is of special value in conditions brought on by shock, cold (north, north-east or east) winds, excessive heat or excessive cold. Its symptoms tend to centre on the chest.

**Colic** – *seek veterinary help promptly but give:*

*Colocynth* – the typical cramping pains of this condition are susceptible to this remedy. It may help prior to veterinary assistance arriving.

*While homeopathy will almost always help colic cases, it will not prevent the need for surgery in certain cases.*

## Collapse

*Aconite* – as always, it is of great value in sudden onset conditions.

*Carbo veg.* – this is known as the 'corpse reviver', based on its well-tried value in extreme collapse. There is usually air-hunger and cyanosis in suitable patients.

*Call the vet.*

## Conjunctivitis

*Aconite* – if acute onset, with watery discharge, esp. if brought on by cold north-east wind.

*Euphrasia* – if acute, worse in blustery weather. This remedy will usually help **any** eye complaint to an extent. The remedy can also make a very useful eye lotion.

*Pulsatilla* – if with greenish-yellow discharges.

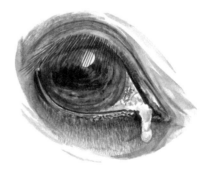

## Corns

*Arnica* – in the acute, initial stages.

*Silica* – if they have become chronic or infected.

## Cough

*Aconite* – if acute and especially if brought on by cold wind.

*Drosera* – if 'deep' and sonorous.

*Hepar sulph.* – if expectoration contains pus.

*Call vet if worried – if the horse is suffering from COPD, then homeopathic veterinary help will be necessary.*

## Cracked hooves

*Graphites* – if accompanied by a tendency to poor healing of skin wounds.

*Silica* – if horn quality is poor and there is a tendency to white line separation or abscess.

*This is a complex condition and the author would usually support prescriptions with a mixture of herbs, specially formulated for the patient, in order to aid correct nutrition. The author usually liaises with the farrier too. The author avoids any supplements containing animal products.*

## Curb

*Ruta grav.* – this remedy helps to heal ligament or tendon damage of all types.

*Call vet if worried.*

## Cuts

*Calendula lotion* – applied to the wound, this will aid healing and reduce sepsis. Many cuts do not need stitching, depending upon size, shape and location.

*Staphisagria* – this medicine will usually speed mental and physical recovery.

## Diarrhoea

*Arsen. alb.* – if foul smelling.

*Nux vom.* – if from overeating.

*Call vet if worried, as it can be a sign of more serious disease.*

## Excitement

*Pulsatilla* – if natural exuberance in a filly.

*Aconite* – if it exceeds normality.

*Argent. nit.* – if accompanied by diarrhoea.

# Treatment guide cont.

## Fear

*Aconite* – if the result of a sudden shock or fright.

*Lycopodium* – if in anticipation of an 'ordeal' or 'challenge'.

## Foot abscess/infected foot

*Ledum* – if a hoof penetration has occurred, in order to try to prevent abscessation.

*Hepar sulph.* – in early and very painful stages.

*Silica* – if more of a chronic nature, perhaps with hoof crumbling or distortion.

## Foot injury

*Hypericum* – for injuries to the foot which are not abscesses or puncture wounds.

## Foreign body

*Silica* – this remedy has an unrivalled reputation for stimulating the necessary abscessation and rejection of the offending item, which may be, for example, a thorn, a grass seed or a splinter.

## Grazes – see Abrasions

## Haematoma

*Arnica* – for its beneficial effects on all bruising-type conditions.

*Hamamelis* – to help reduce bleeding and to speed resolution of the swelling.

## Heat stress

*Aconite* – always useful in sudden and stress-related conditions.

*Glonoinium* – a remedy very well suited to rebalancing the heat-stressed or heat-stroke horse.

## Hysteria

*Ignatia* – this is the remedy most likely to help in cases of hysteria, but there is usually respiratory difficulty and some shock or bereavement behind the problem.

## Infected foot – see Foot abscess

## Injury

*Arnica* – always give Arnica, then look up specific injury types, for more direct help.

## Irritability

*Nux vom.* – if there is a lot of stress in the stable yard or work.

*Sepia* – if in a crotchety mare.

## Laminitis

• in the acute stages:

*Belladonna* – where there is much heat, pain and pulsation, with a refusal to move.

*Hypericum* – to help with the acute pain.

*Bryonia* – usually helps when there is unwillingness to move and less acute symptoms.

• in the chronic stages:

*This calls for experienced veterinary help, since so much can be done for such cases homeopathically, but Graphites may help.*

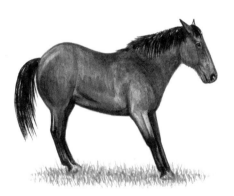

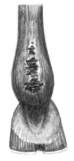
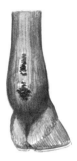

## Mud fever

*Graphites* – sticky moist discharges. If this fails, a homeopathic vet may help, as it can be a very complex condition.

## Muscle injury

*Arnica* – as in the case of any injury or bruise.

*Rhus tox.* – can be of special help to injured muscles, in addition to Arnica.

## Nervousness/anxiety

*Argent. nit.* – if leads to diarrhoea.

*Arsen. alb.* – if panic.

*Lycopodium* – if general anxiety prior to 'ordeal' but performs well.

*Pulsatilla* – if generally timid but friendly.

*Silica* – if very timid, fearful and submissive.

# Treatment guide cont.

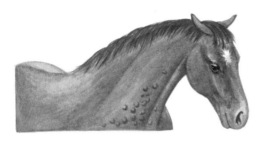

## Nettle rash/urticaria

*Apis mel.* – if the lesions are soothed by cold bathing or applications.

*Urtica* – if the lesions are soothed by warm bathing or applications.

## Oedema (accumulation of fluid)

*Apis mel.* – this is commonly the remedy of choice.

*If generalised, this may herald serious disease.*

## Panic

*Aconite* – usually promptly restores harmony to the overwrought patient.

## Photosensitivity – see Sunburn

## Pining/bereavement

*Ignatia* – if tending towards hysteria.

*Nat. mur.* – if tending towards moroseness and looking withdrawn.

## Proud flesh – see Warts

## Puncture wounds

*Ledum* – in order to try to prevent infection, tetanus or abscessation.

*Hepar sulph.* – in early and very painful stages of septic infection.

## Ringworm

*Bacillinum* – this remedy will often help.

*The author recommends consulting a homeopathic vet, since this is a complex and infectious disease, which can spread to humans too. Prompt, effective treatment and control may not be achieved with a single remedy.*

## Saddle sores

*Arnica* – internal treatment.

*Hypericum and Calendula lotion* – topical treatment.

*This condition should not arise with proper saddling, so immediate remedial measures are necessary, to avoid recurrence. The horse should not be ridden until sores are completely healed.*

## Sarcoids – see Warts

## Separation anxiety

*Arsen. alb.* – will usually help the horse who runs about frantically and is generally very restless under such circumstances.

## Stings

*Apis mel.* – if swollen.

*Cantharis* – if blistered.

*Urtica* – if urticarial (nettle-rash type) reaction.

## Splints

*Silica* – if no complications.

*Arnica* – in early stages.

## Sunburn/photosensitivity

*Hypericum* – should both ease the pain and aid healing.

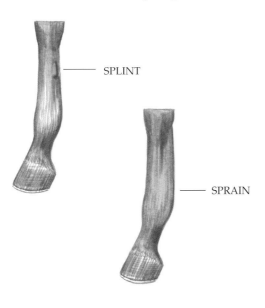

SPLINT

SPRAIN

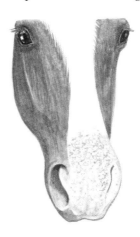

## Surgery

*Arnica* – to minimise the effects of bruising or infection.

*Staphisagria* – this medicine will usually speed mental and physical recovery.

*Calendula lotion* – used topically on the wound, this will aid healing and reduce sepsis.

*Hepar sulph.* – if the wound becomes infected/septic.

## Sprains

*Ruta grav.* – this remedy helps to heal ligament or tendon damage of all types.

*Apis mel.* – in addition, if there is oedematous swelling.

*Call vet if worried.*

# Treatment guide cont.

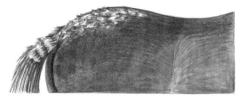

## Sweet itch

*Apis mel.* – will suit the hot, painful and swollen lesions sometimes seen.

*Graphites* – will suit the fat and lazy pony, with a very itchy skin and clear, sticky discharges from the lesions.

*This complex condition may require help from a homeopathic vet.*

## Tail injury

*Hypericum* – in order to help preserve or heal nerves and to reduce pain.

## Tendon injury

*Ruta grav.* – this remedy helps to heal ligament or tendon damage of all types.

*Call vet if worried.*

## Thrush

*Hypericum/Calendula lotion* – bathe the area liberally and often, after properly cleaning out diseased tissue.

## Urticaria – see Nettle rash

## Warts/sarcoids/proud flesh

*Thuja* – first-line remedy for these types of lesion.

*The author warns, however, that Thuja will not be correct for all cases and **should not be given for longer than a week** without veterinary advice and support.*

## Windgalls

*Apis mel.* – helps simple windgalls; if caused by injury, call a vet.

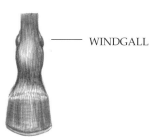

WINDGALL

## Wounds (see also Abrasions/grazes)

*Calendula lotion* – used topically this will aid healing and reduce sepsis. Many wounds do not need stitching, depending upon size, shape and location.

*Hepar sulph.* – if infected/septic.

*Staphisagria* – this medicine will usually speed mental and physical recovery.

# The remedies

**Aconite** (Aconitum napellus) – The characteristic fields of action for this medicine are fear, anxiety, terror, excitement, fevers of sudden onset, conjunctivitis of sudden onset, acute inflammatory reactions and any sudden conditions resulting from cold, dry winds.

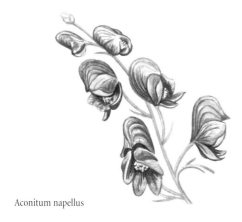

Aconitum napellus

**Apis mel.** (Apis mellifica) – This is a valuable medicine in cases of shiny oedematous (puffy) swellings which retain an impression when indented. Patients usually desire open air and sometimes makes this desire very obvious, particularly those with accumulation of fluid. Helps to clear oedema from joints, tendon sheaths and bursae and can help with urticaria or swollen skin. Improved by cool applications.

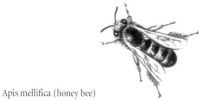

Apis mellifica (honey bee)

**Argent. nit.** (Argentum nitricum) – There is a picture, in this medicine, of anticipatory anxiety and an impatient, impulsive, possibly angry mentality. The horse is prone to conjunctivitis. Diarrhoea can occur with fear or with sweetened, hard feed and usually occurs just after eating.

**Arnica** (Arnica montana) – This is a medicine everyone should have in the household and stable. It is the ultimate *first remedy* for any case of **injury, shock** or **surgery**. Such a remedy is called a vulnerary. You can also use it to prevent or help problems from overexertion. It can be used years after an injury, to lessen persistent after-effects. It is a powerful remedy to combat sepsis of wounds. It can also be used in lotions and ointments. The sooner it is used after an injury, the better is its effect. It is not recommended for *topical* treatment of open wounds. It can be used with other injury remedies where applicable.

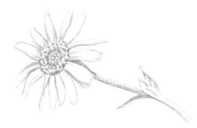

Arnica montana

**Arsen. alb.** (Arsenicum album) – Think of Arsenicum in cases of anxiety or restlessness. Discharges from the eyes and nose are usually acrid and burning. Violent diarrhoea is another possible characteristic of Arsenicum, especially after ingestion of spoilt food. There is often a thirst for frequent small drinks. The skin may be itchy, dry and scaly, with much scurf. Allergic asthmatic conditions often respond well. Symptoms are worse for cold and wet and better for warmth, and are usually worse around midnight.

# The remedies cont.

**Bacillinum** (Bacillinum) – This is a nosode, made from tuberculosis material. It should therefore only be used under the supervision of a veterinary surgeon who is trained in homeopathy. It suits lesions which turn grey and crusty, therefore being of value in some cases of ringworm in horses.

**Belladonna** (Atropa belladonna) – This is a remedy suited to sudden onset conditions, usually with dramatic symptoms. Think of it in cases of fever, abscessation, inflammation, convulsions or violent temper. Symptoms are worse for noise, jarring or touch and are better for warmth and peaceful surroundings, with subdued light.

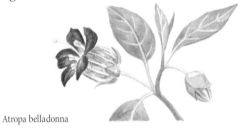

Atropa belladonna

**Bryonia** (Bryonia alba) – Bryonia is an important rheumatism and arthritis remedy. Symptoms are worse for movement and better for rest, so the animal prefers to be still (see also Rhus tox.). A dry cough, diarrhoea (particularly after eating fallen fruit), colic and large thirst are all indications for Bryonia.

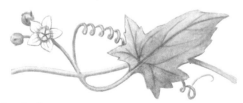

Bryonia alba

**Calc. fluor.** (Calcarea fluorica) – This compound of calcium and fluorine has its special field of action in cases where hard swellings are a feature. Glandular swellings, mammary growths, deforming arthritis and bony malnutrition of foals, are examples. It also helps in controlling adhesions after abdominal surgery. Symptoms are worse for damp weather and at rest but are better for warmth and a little exercise. It is a remedy commonly considered in bone development problems.

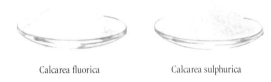

Calcarea fluorica                Calcarea sulphurica

**Calc. sulph.** (Calcarea sulphurica) – This is suited to the treatment of discharging, slow-healing, purulent (involving pus) lesions. Yellowish discharges are usual. As with Silica, it also helps chronic catarrh but of a yellowish nature.

**Calendula** (Calendula officinalis) – Customarily used mainly as a topical lotion or cream, it is a great healing remedy, speeding healing of abrasions, reducing suppuration and aiding first-time healing of wounds.

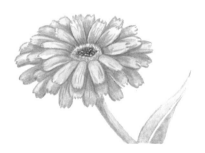

Calendula officinalis

**Cantharis** (Cantharis vesicatoria) – This medicine is useful in cases of sore skin with a blistering rash (e.g. after burns). It is also the first-choice remedy for the horse which shows a frequent urge to pass urine, passing only small quantities but with an empty bladder (beware of those with similar symptoms but with a full bladder – they may be obstructed). There is apparent pain on urination and there may be blood.

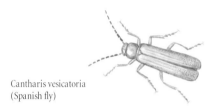

Cantharis vesicatoria
(Spanish fly)

**Carbo veg.** (Carbo vegetabilis) – This is found to be especially helpful in cases of colicky diarrhoea with flatulence, usually worse after food. It is to be recommended where there is collapse or near-collapse with a cold body and warm head. The patient desires open air. Prostration after the least exertion features in its properties and it is referred to as the 'homeopathic corpse reviver', so give it even when the patient is thought to be near to death. When the vital force is nearly totally extinguished it has been known to produce a reversal of the downward trend. It is naturally assumed that a patient this ill is under veterinary care, however.

**Causticum** (Causticum hahnemannii) – This is primarily a rheumatic remedy, most applicable when pains are better for warmth. Also in its sphere are easily bleeding warts, intertrigo (rawness in folds of skin) and scars that redden easily. It is a useful 'old horse' remedy, when they show signs of weakness, contracture of tendons, etc. Problems are worse for cold, dry conditions and for movement. They tend to be better in warm, humid conditions.

**Colocynth** (Citrullus colocynthis) – Colic is the byword for this medicine. In typical cases, the back is hunched and limbs pulled up. There is usually much agitation and evidence of pain coming in spasms. The patient grinds its teeth and is very sensitive to noise. All deep, severe pains may be helped, wherever they are in the body (e.g. hip pain).

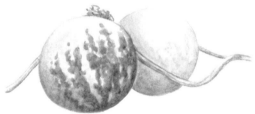

Citrullus colocynthis

**Drosera** (Drosera rotundifolia) – Acting predominantly on the respiratory system, particularly when there is a cough which occurs in paroxysms and is very deep-sounding, this medicine is a frequent visitor to large horse yards. The cough is usually worse in the hours of darkness.

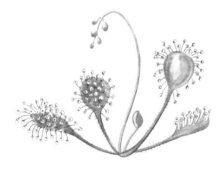

Drosera rotundifolia

# The remedies cont.

**Euphrasia** (Euphrasia officinalis) – This is mainly an eye remedy, suiting symptoms of conjunctivitis, sensitivity to bright light and watery discharge from eyes and nose. Symptoms are worse for wind, warmth and bright light and are better for subdued light. It is used internally or in the form of eye drops. The plant's familiar name is 'eye-bright'.

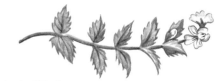

Euphrasia officinalis

**Glonoinium** (Glonoinium) – This remedy is a powerful heart treatment but its special sphere of activity, and therefore its main source of interest to the reader, is in its ability to counter the effects of heat stroke and heat stress.

**Graphites** (Graphites) – Mostly this is a skin remedy, useful in cases exhibiting cracked skin with a sticky exudate, especially in the bends of the limbs. Constitutionally, patients are generally fat, chilly types with a tendency to constipation. Hoof condition tends to be poor in suitable patients.

**Hamamelis** (Hamamelis virginica) – Seeping dark haemorrhages, haematomata, venous pooling or leakage of venous blood fit the picture of this remedy.

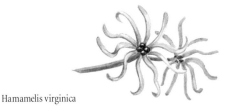

Hamamelis virginica

**Hepar sulph.** (Hepar sulphuris) – This has been called the 'homeopathic antibiotic' but, in reality, there is no such thing – its amazing ability to help the patient fight off septic-type infections is the reason. It is a very important remedy in suppurative conditions. It is useful either as a preventive or curative treatment in septic injury. Pus in the eyes also responds. All septic conditions should remind one of this remedy, including infected wounds, whether of surgical or accidental origin.

**Hypericum** (Hypericum perforatum) – This medicine's ability to help in painful conditions has earned it the nickname of the 'homeopathic painkiller'. Use it in cases of injury to extremities where nerve endings abound, particularly toe or tail injuries. Post-operative pain, spinal injury, lacerated wounds and puncture wounds all may show much-needed relief from this remedy. It also has reputed anti-tetanus properties.

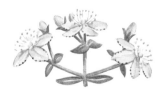

Hypericum perforatum

**Ignatia** (Ignatia amara) – Well known as a remedy for bereavement, it is very powerful in circumstances where pining and grief are uppermost. Use after any mental shock, death of an owner (or close companion) or other such situations. Its effects have shown up in unexpected ways, including skin conditions, where one supposes (sometimes in retrospect) that pining or grief may be involved in the cause. Horses upset by separation can often be helped by this remedy. There is a tendency to hysteria in suitable patients.

**Lachesis** (Lachesis muta) – Centring its actions on the throat it also suits mostly left-sided complaints of the nervous and vascular systems and of the skin. It is a constitutional remedy and thus affects all parts of the body, but its main areas of acute usage are paralysis, haemorrhage, haematoma, hurried manner and restlessness, with a tendency to suspicion and hyper-reactivity. It may be useful in female hormonal problems, where the symptoms fit this picture and especially if the left ovary is involved.

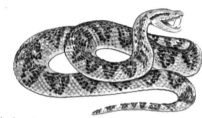

Lachesis muta

**Ledum** (Ledum palustre) – Like Hypericum, Ledum has reputed but unproven anti-tetanus properties. It is the first-choice remedy for puncture wounds. It helps them to heal properly, i.e. from the bottom upwards. In more complex homeopathy, it also has uses for arthritic pain in small joints which are worse for heat or warmth. Nail injuries in the foot call for this remedy, but it does not remove the need for adequate paring of the sole.

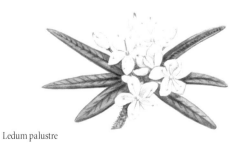

Ledum palustre

**Lycopodium** (Lycopodium clavatum) – Respiratory, digestive, hepatic (liver) and urinary conditions suggest Lycopodium. Marked but easily-satisfied hunger is a consistent symptom. Difficulty with defaecation or the presence of urinary stones can also be helped. Symptoms are better for cold or motion and are worse for heat.

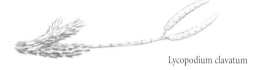

Lycopodium clavatum

**Nat. mur.** (Natrum muriaticum) – A deep-acting remedy, this treats the long-term effects of grief, especially in morose horses. Other symptoms which can respond are persistent 'nose clearing', thin nasal discharge, watery eyes and crusty skin lesions, particularly in the bends of the limbs. The patient is usually very chilly but symptoms are worse for heat and warmth and are better for open air.

**Nux vom.** (Nux vomica) – This is most suited to horses who are stressed by a heavy training programme and who are fed a lot of grain. Digestive disturbances following unsuitable food, constipation (sometimes diarrhoea) after overeating, irritable temperament, sensitivity to noise, muscular spasm and stuffed-up nose are all in the realm of Nux vomica. Symptoms are worse for noise and better for rest or in damp weather. The morning is usually when symptoms are at their worst.

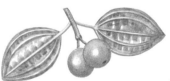

Nux vomica

# The remedies cont.

**Pulsatilla** (Pulsatilla nigricans) – Paradox and variability are the themes of this medicine. It suits an animal (usually female) of shy or retiring disposition. The patient is, however, a friendly type. Most symptoms are very variable. Intermittent diarrhoea, faddy appetite which comes and goes, and (usually) very little thirst are all associated with Pulsatilla. It has proved useful in many (particularly female) hormonal problems. The Pulsatilla patient is usually quite cheerful but easily dispirited. Muco-purulent (mucus and pus) discharges are bland and greenish-yellow. There can be, paradoxically, a weak pulse with fever.

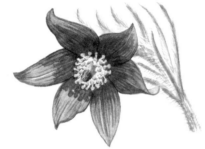

Pulsatilla nigricans

**Rhus tox.** (Rhus toxicodendron) – This medicine is mainly of use in the skin and musculoskeletal systems. The skin shows small red pimples or small blisters. The rheumatic/arthritic symptoms are its greatest sphere of success, where it is the first choice remedy for symptoms that are worse for cold, wet conditions and worse

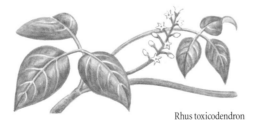

Rhus toxicodendron

for first movement after rest or confinement. Conditions are better for continued movement and for warmth. Excessive exercise again produces a worsening. Where there is trauma to muscles, think of this medicine.

**Ruta grav.** (Ruta graveolens) – Think of this remedy in connection with sprains and dislocations and you will understand much of its properties. Where any tendon, ligament, joint or bone is injured turn to Ruta. It also helps rheumatic symptoms which are similar to Rhus, and it can be used in conjunction with Rhus.

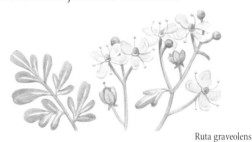

Ruta graveolens

**Sepia** (Sepia officinalis) – A constitutional remedy, Sepia is used mostly, like Pulsatilla, in the treatment of female ailments. Moody conditions arising from hormonal problems (e.g. bad-tempered behaviour around time of seasons) are its great sphere of action, along with loss of tone or infection of the womb and pelvic organs. The patient tends to indifference. Pulsatilla types can often 'age' into Sepia types.

Sepia officinalis (cuttlefish)

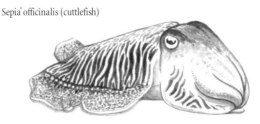

**Silica** (Silica) – Usually a very shy, retiring and chilly animal, reluctant to face ordeals, typifies the mental side of Silica. Chronic inflammatory conditions (e.g. sinus infection), foreign bodies (e.g. blackthorns in the tissues), fragments of bone after injury and septic conditions which refuse to suppurate are all in Silica's province. Typical suitable lesions repeatedly burst, leak pink fluid or pus, and reseal.

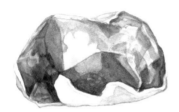

Silica

**Staphisagria** (Delphinium staphisagria) – Known mostly as a resentment remedy, Staphisagria is frequently used for horses who appear to have had their noses 'put out of joint' psychologically. They may feel usurped by a new arrival into the establishment or may have been abused. Post-operative and accidental trauma problems can be helped, especially if there are lacerations or stretched orifices.

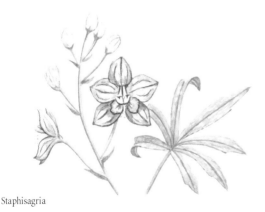

Staphisagria

**Symphytum** (Symphytum officinale) – Known also as comfrey or 'knitbone,' it has an unsurpassed reputation in the speeding and regulation of bone healing. Use it also in injuries to the eye area (orbit) and to the fibrous eyeball itself.

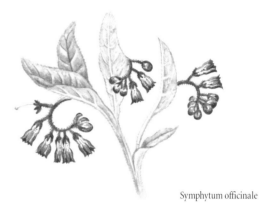

Symphytum officinale

**Thuja** (Thuja occidentalis) – This remedy is the most common treatment for warts, particularly of the pedunculated or 'fig' type. It has an application in some sarcoid cases and in the treatment of adverse reactions to vaccination, an important area which this little book has not been able to consider.

**Urtica** (Urtica urens) – This is of great value in the treatment of the so-called 'urticarial' or 'nettle' rash. Suitable allergic, patchy swellings of the skin are improved by warm applications and aggravated by cold water. Burns (before blistering) and similar lesions respond well. In high potency it promotes milk flow in mares, while in very low potency it has a reputation for helping mammary glands to 'dry up', as may be needed at weaning or if a foal should die at foot. (Refer also to Apis mel.).

# General care

However well chosen the homeopathic medicine, better results can always be achieved by paying attention to other factors which can directly affect your horse's health or healing. The main examples are:

- Healthy diet (the author advises caution with molasses and other additives).

- Pure supplements (buy only when needed) containing no ingredients of animal origin. If used, these should be integrated properly with feeding and medical regimes.

- Pasture management, especially with regard to caution with fertilisers and chemicals.

- Detailed attention to comfortable and well-fitted saddles and tack, good and properly balanced shoeing, well-attended teeth, proper back care, good general management and care and, of course, careful and considerate handling and riding.

This is the basis of properly applied holistic medicine; your horse's all-round welfare should be your major concern. Besides the health benefits, a well-cared-for horse will pay you dividends in performance, pleasure and longevity.

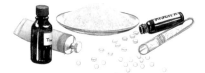

# Obtaining homeopathic remedies and help

A limited range of commonly used homeopathic medicines is now available in many health shops, pharmacies, feed merchants, etc. The range will cover most first-aid applications and the medicines are just as suitable for humans as for any other species.

In the rare circumstance of a more unusual remedy being required, a homeopathic veterinary surgeon will usually be able to supply it. Alternatively it may be available via mail-order from specialist homeopathic pharmacies.

**In the UK** The British Association of Homeopathic Veterinary Surgeons (BAHVS) holds a regularly updated list of homeopathic vets, which is obtainable by sending a self-addressed, stamped envelope marked 'HORSES' to:
BAHVS, c/o The Alternative Veterinary Medicine Centre, Chinham House, Stanford in the Vale, Oxon, SN7 8NQ

**In the USA**, contact:
The American Holistic Veterinary Medical Association, 2214 Old Emmorton Road, Bel Air, MD 21015

**For other countries**, The International Association for Veterinary Homeopathy can help:
General Secretary IAVH, Sonnhaldenstr. 24, CH – 8370 Sirnach, Switzerland